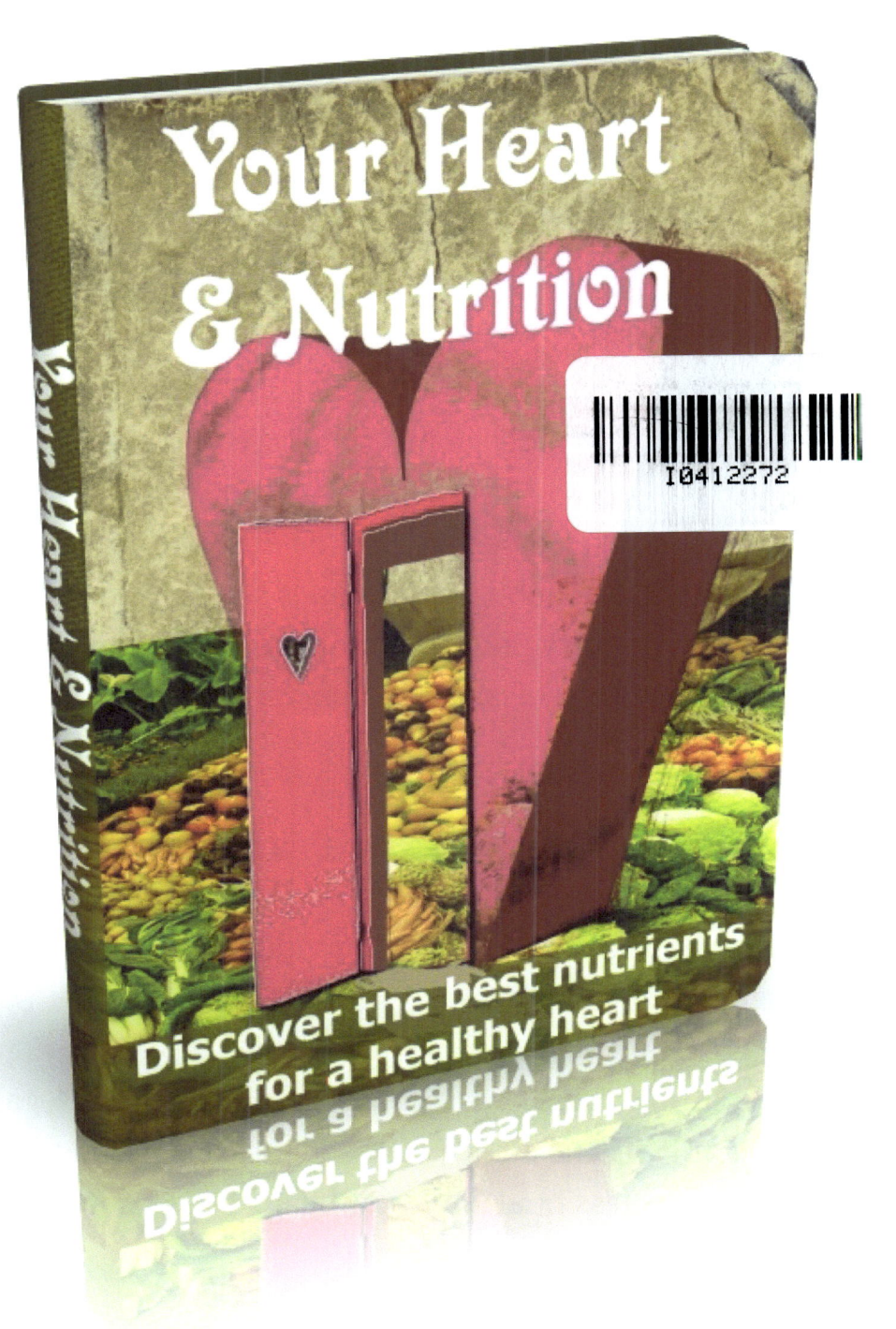

# Your Heart & Nutrition

Discover the best nutrients for a healthy heart

# Terms and Conditions

## LEGAL NOTICE

# Table Of Contents

# Foreword

There is a growing number of fatalities that are attributed heart diseases and thus the need arises to all humans to be well informed and concerned with this growing unhealthy state. There are several changes that can be made in an individual's life to try and control this condition from occurring in one's lifetime. Get all the info you need here.

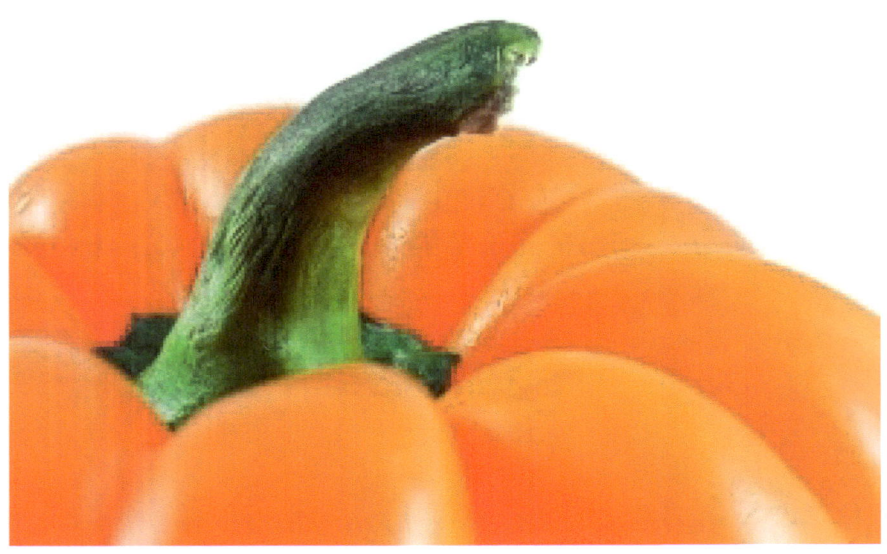

### *Your Heart & Nutrition*
Discover the best nutrients for a healthy heart

# Chapter 1:

## *Preventive Steps To Lower Your Risk Of Heart Disease*

# Synopsis

The following are some of the steps that can be taken to ensure the possibility of a heart disease condition from occurring:

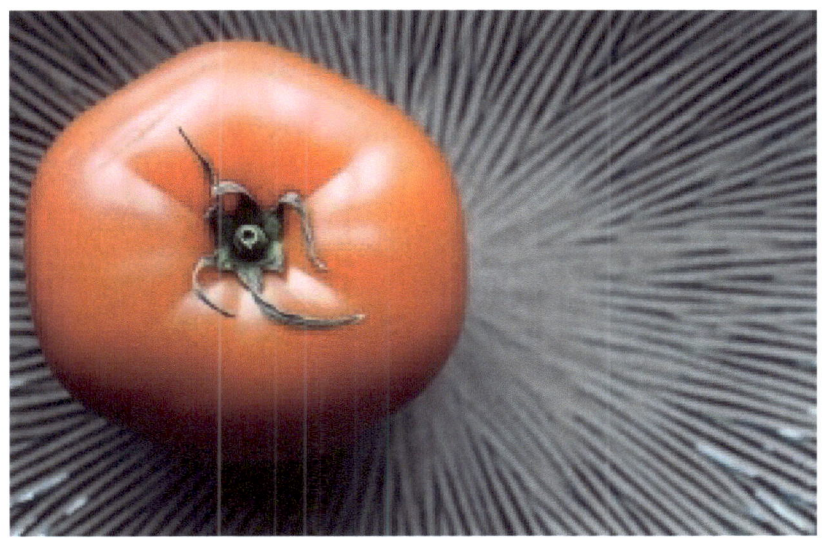

# The Basics

The most obvious and often disregarded rule would be to not smoke as this is not only a bad habit to form it is also a deadly one. Records have shown that those who have made the conscious effort to stop smoking have been able to bring down and even eliminate their chances of suffering from heart diseases.

Keeping the cholesterol levels low and manageable is also another important exercise to consider as the high blood cholesterol is a condition that increases the risks of developing coronary heart disease.

This is caused by the narrowing of the arteries thus inhibiting the flow of blood to the heart. Ideally the cholesterol levels should be below 200mg/dl; LDL cholesterol below 130mg/dl and HLD above 35mg/dl.

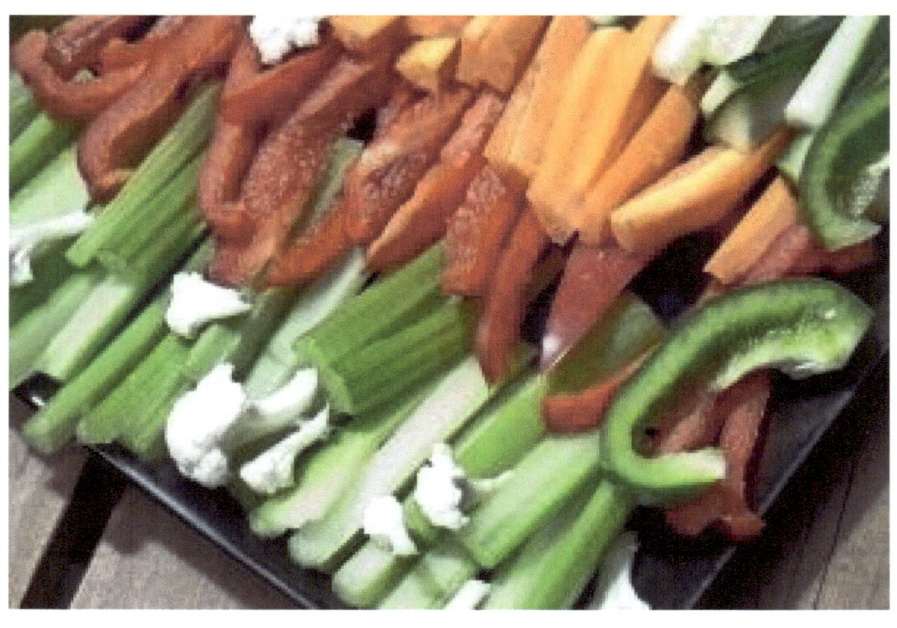

# Chapter 2:

## *Role Of Nutrition In Heart Disease Treatment*

# Synopsis

There are several issues related or connected to the occurrences of the heart disease condition in an individual and having all the necessary facts to help make the right decisions, when it comes to medically prescribed supplements, nutrition and just the general diet should be given due consideration.

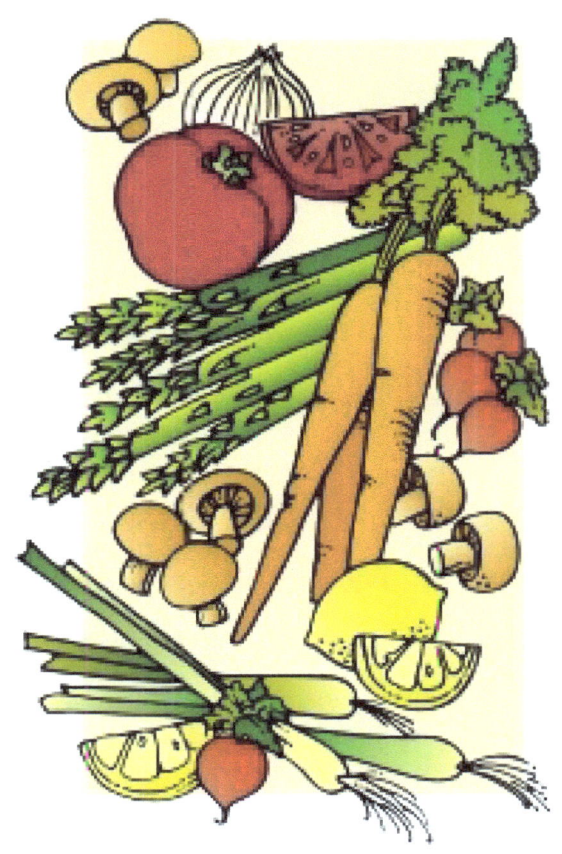

# How It Works

It has been noted that a lot of the less than desirable heart conditions are usually brought on by the lack of proper nutrition in the diet plan of an individual.

Therefore when taking precautions to avoid this disease the nutritional overall content in the diet plan accompanied with the needed medical prescriptions, if needed, should be well balanced. Some of the points that should be noted when designing such a diet plan would be as follows:

The avoidance of processed foods should be one of the priorities given as these foods can cause some nutrition intakes to become useless to the overall body's benefit.

These foods often come with a high content of sodium which usually reacts in a counterproductive manner in the body's system.

These may include salad dressings, frozen dinner which were originally touted as being nutritious, peanut butter and many other supposedly healthy additions to the diet plan.

Keeping alcohol consumption to a minimal is also another important practice to consider, as it often interferes with the nutritional balance in the diet plan and causes a lot of good properties in the plan to be nullified.

Potassium supplements are often encouraged to be included in the nutritional diet plan, however items such as cheese and nuts should be taken in moderation.

The combination of L-carnitine, Coenzyme Q10, Magnesium and Vitamin E or otherwise known as the CCME combination has often been used as a good nutritional supplement for individual having heart disease conditions.

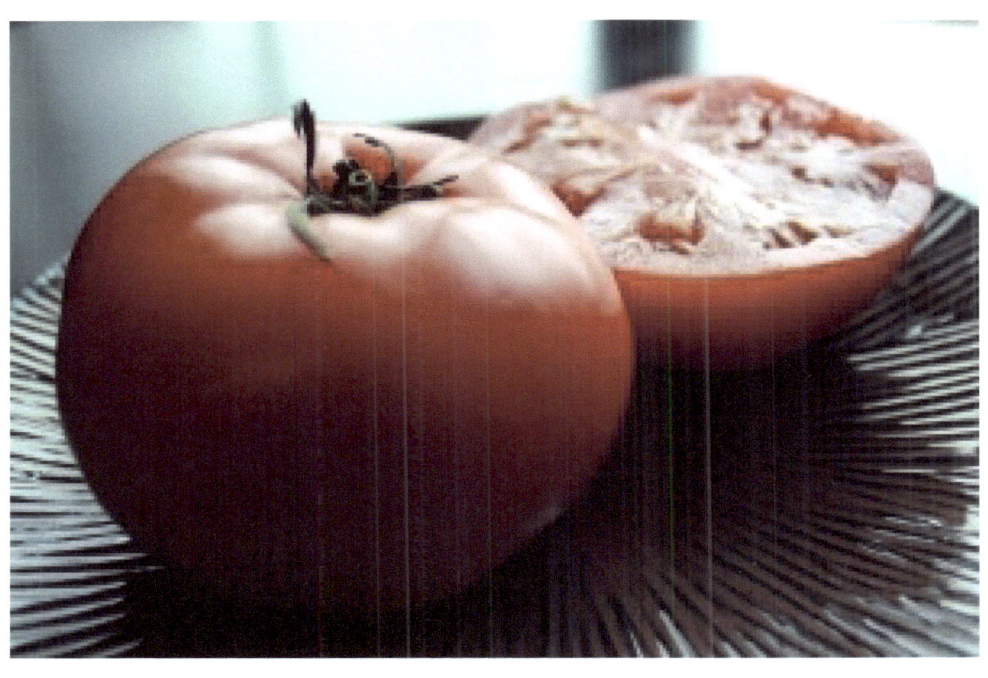

# Chapter 3:
## *The Natural Remedy Enhance Heart Health*

# Synopsis

It is not always necessary to treat heart conditions with medications and medical treatments as sometimes a change of diet and lifestyle can be just as effective. There are many natural remedies that can be tried to control and even reverse the negative heart conditions to a better and healthier condition.

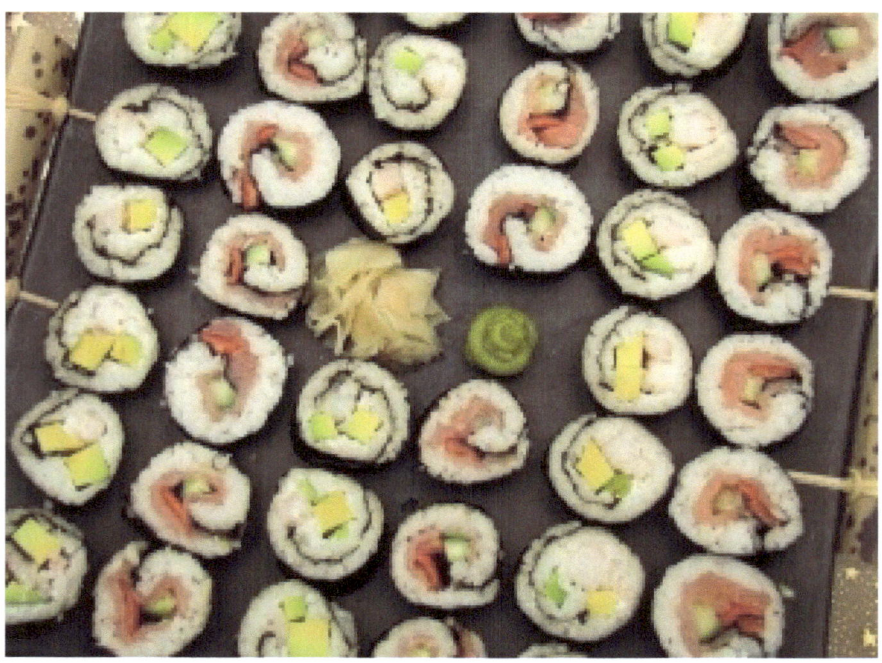

# Enhancements

The following are some of the natural remedies that can be incorporated into the daily diet plan to ensure good heart health conditions:

Consuming bran based products can be beneficial to the overall health of the body system functions. As bran is high in fiber content it will help to keep the cholesterol levels in check, and these can be found in items such as Harley, oats, whole grains which include brown rice and lentils, beans such as kidney beans and black beans.

Olive oil is another highly recommended diet inclusion in the daily regimen of nutritional plans. The monounsaturated sources of which olive oil is prime candidate is definitely a plus to include and can be a substitute when vegetable oils are unavailable.

Peanut butter is also another surprising yet equally beneficial item to be consumed. 2 tablespoons will give the individual a good dose of 1/3 of the daily vitamin E needed. However weight watchers should not be overly enthusiastic with the consumption of this particular food item.

Pecan nuts which are full of magnesium are another hearty friendly nutrient. This can be used in salads or even in baked items as a flavored ingredient to enhance a particular dish. Besides providing the 1/3 daily nutritional needs it is also a very flavor enriched food item.

Wine is often touted as a good item to consume for improved heart conditions, but this should be done in moderation as if not controlled it can and usually does cause the individual to go over board and eventually become an alcoholic.

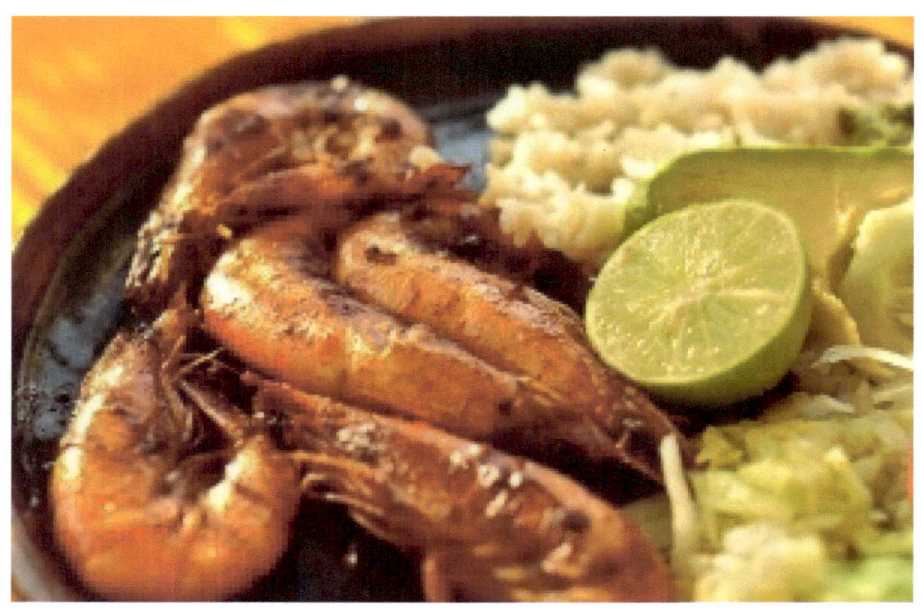

# Chapter 4:

## *Vitamins For A Healthy Heart*

# Synopsis

Through the course of trying to maintain healthy heart conditions, the individual should consider incorporating a good vitamin intake regimen into the daily diet plan thus effectively ensuring a better balance and optimal heat function possibilities. This can be done quite easily with the right vitamin plan in place to cater to this need.

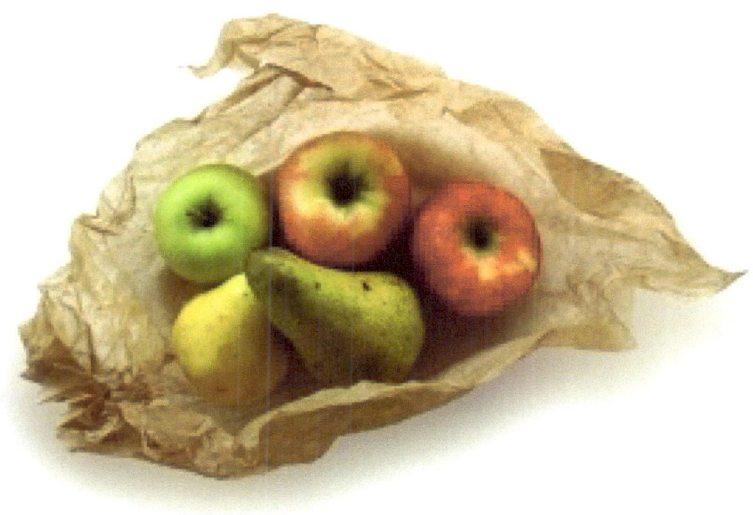

# Vitamins

Most essential heart vitamins should include the use of the vitamin B family elements.

These vitamins serve specific functions and can significantly reduce the risk of developing heart diseases or keeping an already existing condition in check. In some cases it has also played a significant role in elimination the problem altogether.

The vitamin B plays a role in removing homocysteine from the blood which is the main cause of the arteries being damaged. Meat is one good source of this particular vitamin. Vitamin B also contributes to the reduction of cholesterol in the body system as does other vitamins which include vitamin E and C.

Vitamins E and C provide the necessary antioxidants for the heart to function at an optimum level without being stressed with negative complications which are brought on by the inadequate diet and lifestyle plans.

The antioxidants are the elements that remove the toxic byproducts of chemical reactions in the body system as these highly reactive chemicals that circulate within the system are the cause of most of the significant damage done to a healthy heart.

It has also been known to assist in keeping certain cancers and premature aging in check. The vitamin E which is often gotten from the omega 3 oils does have a lot of cardio benefits if taken over a period of time as there is evidence that is can be a good prevention rather than as actual complete cure for the heart disease condition. Thus in the quest to limit the problems that may arise and cause a healthy heart to deteriorate taking this vitamin will certainly help to ensure optimum functioning is prolonged.

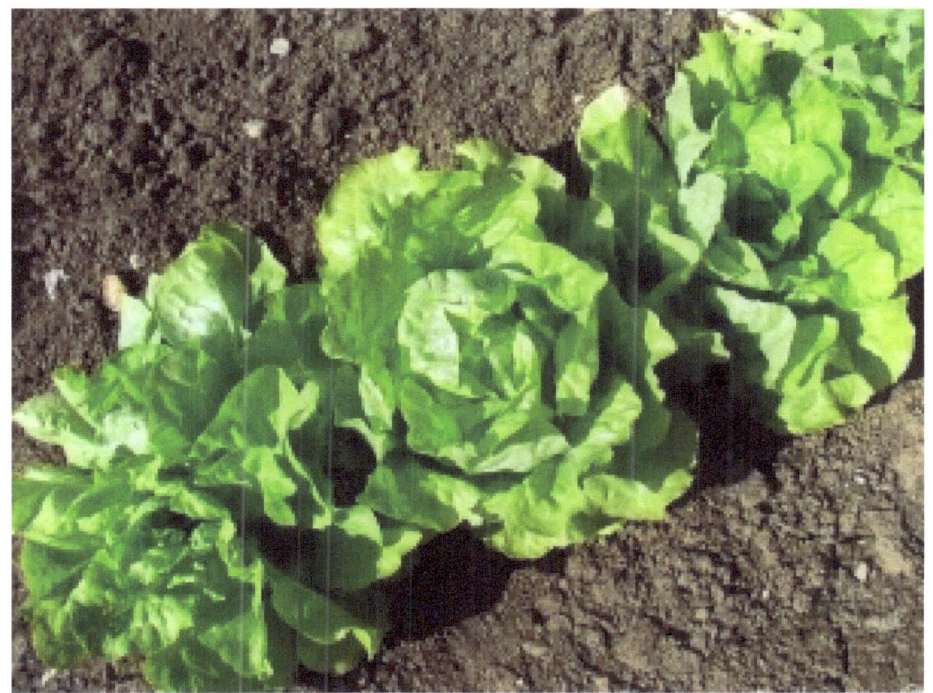

# Chapter 5:
## *Nutritional Supplements Treating Heart Diseases*

# Synopsis

Recently more patients are turning to nutritional supplements to help treat heart disease conditions as opposed to depending on medications. This is due to the fact that for some the nutritional supplements present a better option with fewer side effects as compared to the more conventional medical treatments, thus the popular use.

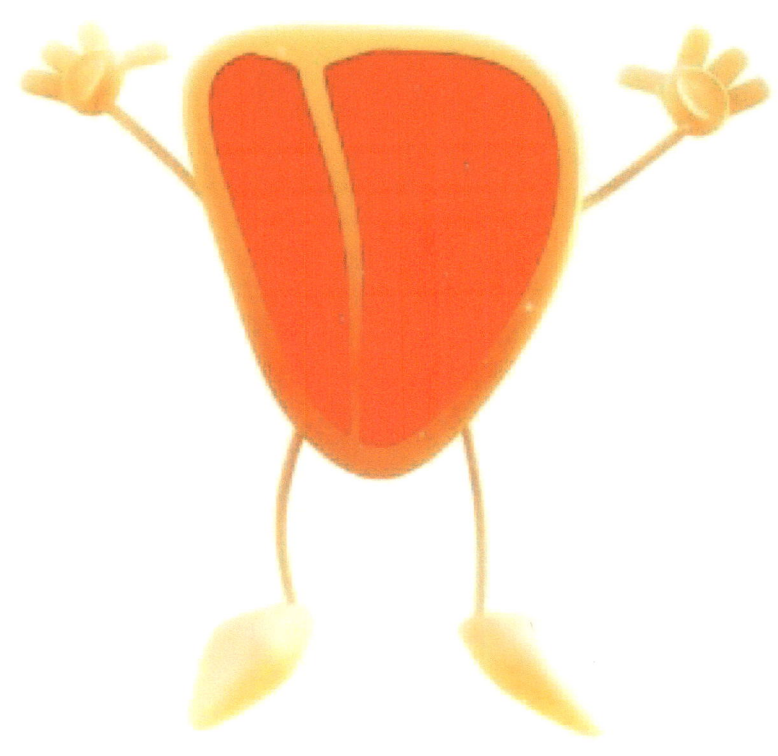

# For Treatment

The following is a guide to the nutritional supplements sources for treating heart disease conditions:

Antioxidant vitamins – these would include the range of vitamins A,C, and E. Taking such vitamins as supplements, for the intention of improving health conditions is something that is becoming very popularly advocated by most medical groups today.

This is done with the added effort to consciously control the blood pressure levels. However it should be noted that the use of such antioxidant vitamins in the form of natural sources from food products should be taken as a whole and not depended upon solely without other more complete and complimenting additions.

Omega-3 fatty acids - this differs with the consumption of the omega-3 fatty acids which is generally accepted as complete supplements in its various forms to be able to combat negative heart conditions or to help create ideally healthy heart conditions.

This supplement which is predominantly derived from the consistent intake of fish does help to give the body system the much needed omega-3 fatty acids to cater to the daily needs of the body.

Folate – this naturally element that is usually found in deep green leafy vegetables, fruits and dried beans is also another important element that ensures good and healthy heart conditions. Vitamin B is the most dominant factor that is derived from this food source. Deficiency of this element will cause the blood vessels to sustain damage and blood clot formations to become rampant which will eventually put a constant strain on the heart condition.

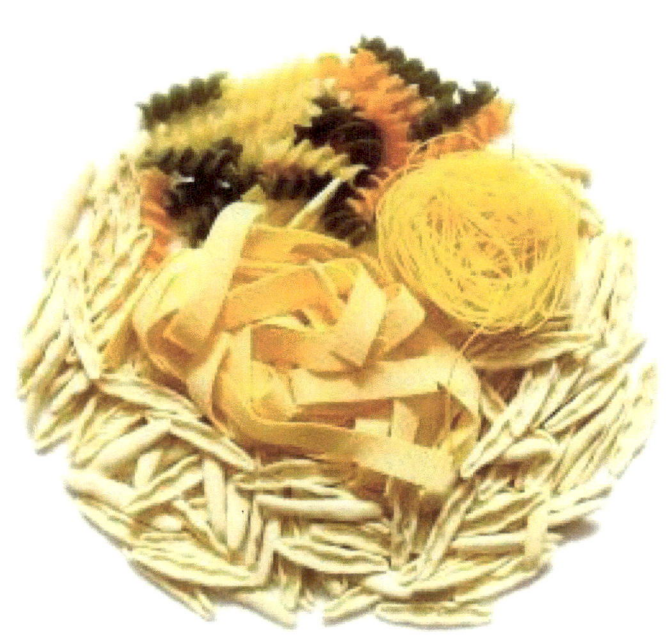

# Chapter 6:

## *Getting Folic Acid For Heart Disease*

# Synopsis

Recent studies have shown that consistent and controlled consumption of the folic acid supplements can reduce the chances of developing heart disease and strike conditions. The folic acid helps to reduce the levels of homocysteine in the body system of an individual.

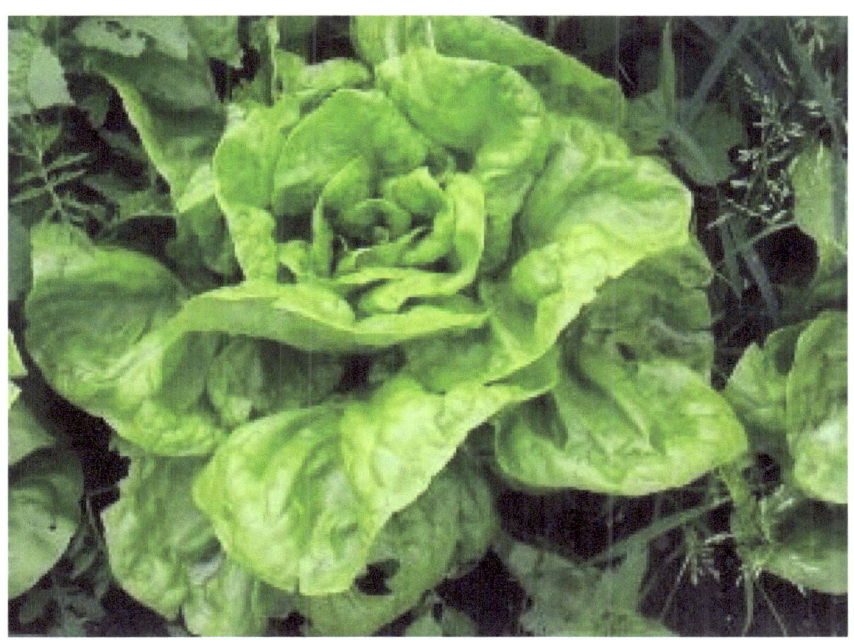

# A Natural Way

The homocysteine is an amino acid in the blood which is often linked to the higher risk of cardiovascular disease and stroke or even peripheral vascular disease.

With the regulated consumption of folic acid it has been found that the homocysteine levels in the blood systems is affectively brought to a more manageable and even healthier level thus eliminating the possibility of causing heart problems.

Being a water soluble vitamin the folate is predominantly found in the vitamin B group. Some ideal dietary sources of folic acid would include dark green leafy vegetables, fortified breakfast cereals, enriched grain products, liver and some other organ meats, lightly cooked beans, peas, nuts and certain seeds, oranges and grapefruits, sprouts, poultry and whole wheat bread.

The folate helps to produce and maintain the new cells and normalize red blood cell conditions. The homocysteine metabolism is kept in check with the maintenance of normal levels of the amino acid.

It has been established that the addition of proper folic acid amount into the daily diet plan has been able to adequately contribute to the reduction in the plasma tHcy concentrations, thus improving endothelial functions. It is generally accepted that the controlled consumption of folic acid in its various form is a relatively inexpensive way of keeping the heart condition and its functions healthy and optimum.

To date most studies conducted have shown that it does have some positive effect on the heart conditions if consumed in a regulated manner. It should be noted that the age of the individual is an important deciding factor in creating the ideal amounts that should be consumed on the daily basis, as an overdose of the folic acid intake can lead to other complications within the body system.

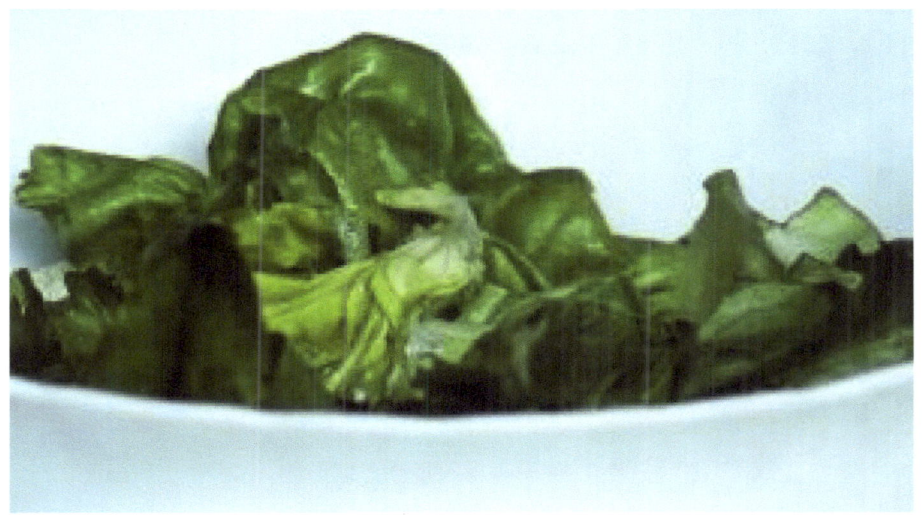

# Chapter 7:

## *Natural Fat Is Good For The Heart*

# Synopsis

It was a previously popular belief that any fats are bad for the human body and in particular the heart. However new research, has since disproven this fact and the current acknowledgement is that certain types of fats are not only good for the human body but are also very much an essential ingredient that contributes to the overall good health conditions.

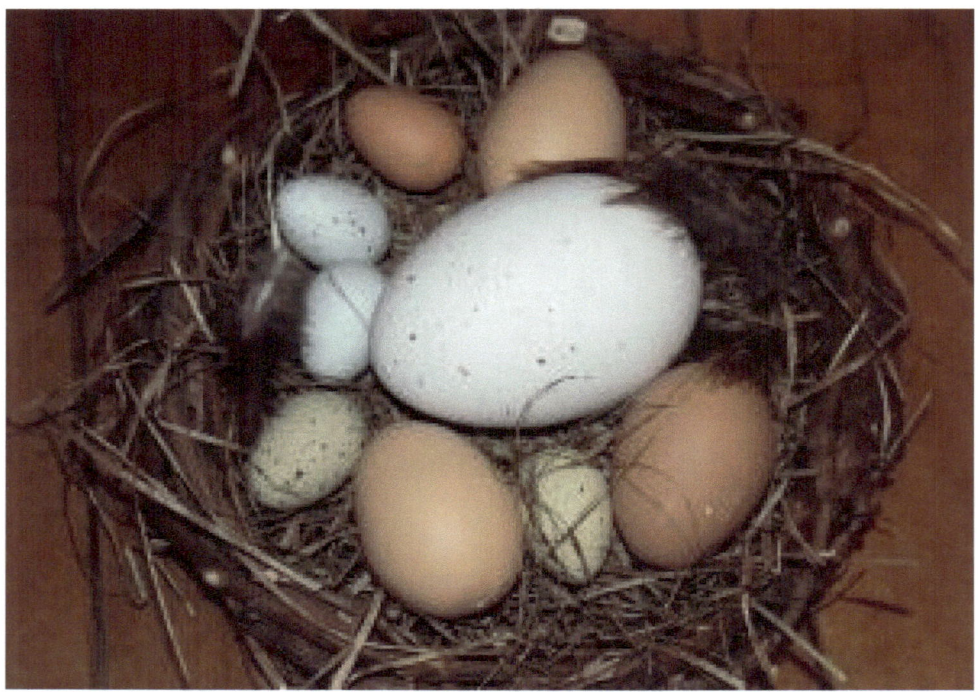

# The Good Fats

Understanding that not all fats are bad is a step in the right direction as it will help the individual to discern the negatives and positives of the different foods consumed. It is a scientifically acknowledged fact that not all fats are alike.

Some are good for health while others can contribute to negative body conditions such as raised blood cholesterol, cardiovascular ill health and unnecessary weight gain.

The following is a list of good fats that should be taken in moderation to ensure optimum heart conditions:

- Omega-3 fatty acids are a type of polyunsaturated fat that can be found in fatty fish such as salmon, herring, sardines and trout. Ideally this should be consumed in three servings of 3 oz each per week. Other ideal sources of omega-3 fatty acids would include flaxseed, walnuts and canola oil.

- As for the polyunsaturated fats in the omega-6 fatty acids group the ideal source of these can be found in vegetable oils such as corn oil, safflower oil, sesame oil. Soybean oil and sunflower oils. There is also the soft margarine source that should be Trans fat free. Walnuts sunflower seeds, pumpkin seeds, sesame seeds, soy as in roasted soy beans, soy nuts butter and tofu are all other alternative sources of omega-6 fatty acids.

- Monounsaturated fats such as vegetable oils, olive oil, canola oil, peanut oil, various types of nuts and avocado are also another source of the good fats for the body.

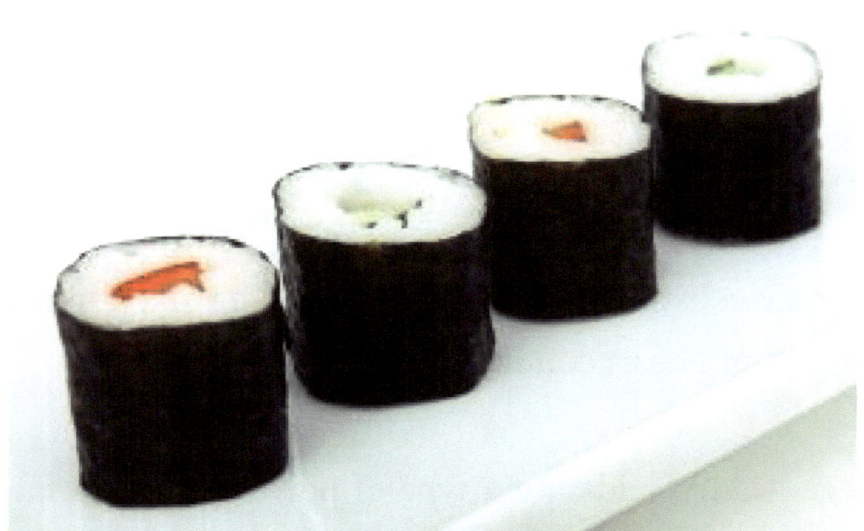

# Wrapping Up

Maintain a healthy body weight is something that all healthy people are conscious on doing on a regular basis. With the ideal weight in place the various body systems do not have to be overworked and stressed to create the ideal functioning systems. Obesity is a dominant contributor to abdominal adiposity which is an important risk factor for cardiovascular disease.

Exercising regularly with an even and not overly stressful regiment would also allow the body to function at its optimum and not be stressed at any time.

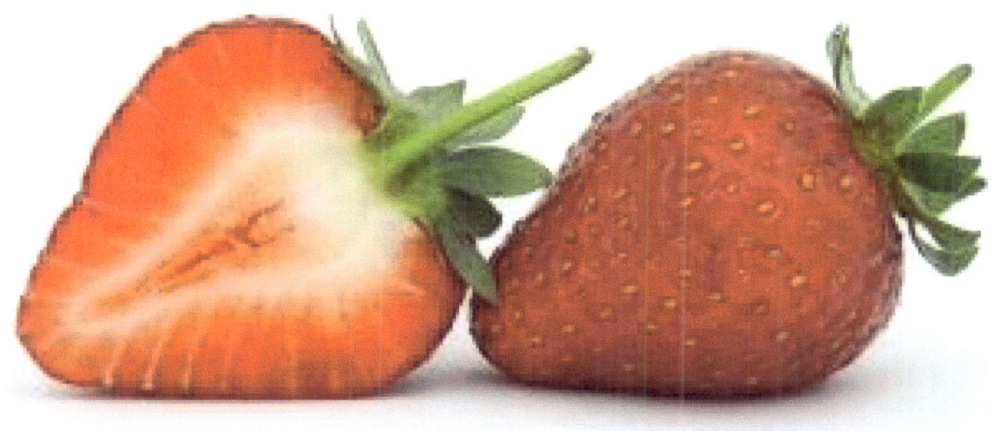